To:

From:

Please consult your physician before undertaking this or any exercise program.

theCouponCollection™

SOURCEBOOKS, INC.
NAPERVILLE, ILLINOIS

a little bit of
yoga

a coupon gift to energize and relax you

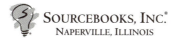

SOURCEBOOKS, INC.®
NAPERVILLE, ILLINOIS

Copyright © 2003 by Sourcebooks, Inc.
Cover and internal design © 2003 by Sourcebooks, Inc.
Cover and internal photo © 2003 Creatas

All rights reserved. No part of this book may be reproduced in any form or by any electronic or mechanical means including information storage and retrieval systems—except in the case of brief quotations embodied in critical articles or reviews—without permission in writing from its publisher, Sourcebooks, Inc.

Published by Sourcebooks, Inc.
P.O. Box 4410, Naperville, Illinois 60567-4410
(630) 961-3900
FAX: (630) 961-2168
www.sourcebooks.com

ISBN 1-4022-0079-X

Printed and bound in the United States of America
DR 10 9 8 7 6 5 4 3 2 1

take a
breath

Take a few gathering breaths
to raise your energy.

Stand straight with toes and ankles touching and hands by your side. As you inhale, raise your arms to the ceiling and touch your palms together over your head. As you exhale, bring your hands into prayer position with palms touching in front of your heart.

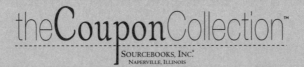

strike a
pose

Become the half moon, stretching both sides of your body and stimulating your creativity.

Stand straight with toes and ankles touching and arms up over your head. Interlace your fingers, with index fingers pointing to the ceiling. Press one hip out and reach your fingertips to the other side of the room. Take a few breaths, then inhale back to standing. Repeat on other side.

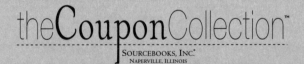

take a
rest

Stand in Mountain pose and ground yourself into the earth.

Stand straight with toes and ankles touching. Arms are at your sides. Feel your feet pressing into the ground, and the crown of your head reaching to the ceiling.

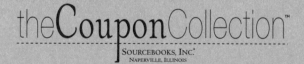

theCouponCollection™

SOURCEBOOKS, INC.
NAPERVILLE, ILLINOIS

take a
breath

Ocean sounding breath will warm you up and make you more flexible.

As you breathe in and out through your nose, gently constrict the back of your throat so you sound as if you were snoring gently.

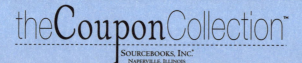

strike a pose

Do a forward bend to bring fresh oxygen to the brain, making you alert and energetic.

As you inhale, circle your arms up over your head. As you exhale, fold forward and reach for your toes. Bend your knees, drape your ribs over your thighs, and relax. Gravity does all the work. When you're ready to come up, bend your knees, tuck your chin, and slowly round up to standing.

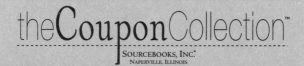

take a
rest

Stand in Mountain Pose and
take three deep breaths.

Stand straight with toes and ankles
touching. Arms are at your sides.
Feel your feet pressing into the ground,
and the crown of your head
reaching to the ceiling.
Breathe deeply.

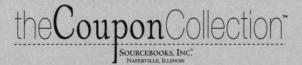

strike a
pose

Take a gentle backbend to stretch
the front of the body.

Inhale your arms up, interlace your fingers with index fingers pointing to the ceiling and gently stretch the front of your body to take a high arch in your upper back. Gaze up at the ceiling. After a few breaths, return to standing.

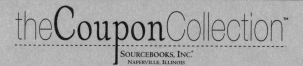

take a
rest

Lie down on the floor and let all your muscles relax for a few breaths.

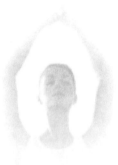

theCouponCollection™

SOURCEBOOKS, INC.
NAPERVILLE, ILLINOIS

strike a
pose

Gently hug your knees to your chest.

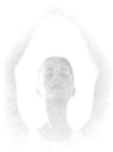

the Coupon Collection™

SOURCEBOOKS, INC.
NAPERVILLE, ILLINOIS

strike a
pose

Use a gentle spinal twist to increase flexibility.

Lying on your back, hug your knees to your chest then open your arms to a T position. Let your knees flop over to one side as you gaze out over the other. Keep your shoulders on the ground and feel a delicious stretch from hip to armpit. Inhale the knees back to center, then exhale to the other side. When you've done both sides equally, inhale the knees back to center.

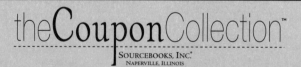

take a
rest

Enjoy the goddess pose—
a resting pose with a little stretch.

Lying on your back, bring the soles of your feet together and let your knees flop open. Increase the stretch by bringing your feet closer to your body, reduce the stretch by moving your feet away. Stretch your arms over your head and clasp your elbows. After a few breaths, release and lie flat.

theCouponCollection™

SOURCEBOOKS, INC.
NAPERVILLE, ILLINOIS

strike a
pose

Sit up for a forward fold,
a lovely stretch for the back of the body.

Sit up straight with your legs stretched out in front of you and your feet flexed. Inhale your arms up, and as you exhale, bend forward and reach for your toes, ankles, or shins. Reach the crown of your head toward your toes and let your shoulder blades glide down your back. After a few breaths, inhale back up to sitting.

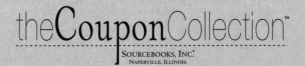

strike a
pose

Stretch the front of the body
in the table pose.

Sitting up, place your feet flat on the floor and your hands behind you on the floor. Inhale and lift your hips toward the ceiling, letting your head fall back. After a few breaths, exhale the hips down to the floor.

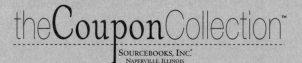

strike a
pose

Do the butterfly, just as you did
when you were a child!

Sit up straight and bring the soles of your feet together. Let your knees flop open. Hold onto your ankles, open your chest, and gaze up at the ceiling. After a few breaths, release your ankles and relax.

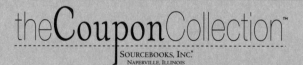

strike a
pose

Open your legs wide and stretch your inner thighs.

Sitting up, open the legs only as far as is comfortable. Gently reach forward, and breathe deeply. When you're ready, sit up.

theCouponCollection™

SOURCEBOOKS, INC.
NAPERVILLE, ILLINOIS

strike a
pose

Take a spinal twist as the perfect way to transition from one posture to another.

Sitting up with your legs straight out in front of you, put your right hand on the outside of your left leg and twist to the left. Put your left hand on the floor behind you. Reach the crown of your head toward the ceiling. When you're ready, release back to center, leading with the chin. Repeat on the other side.

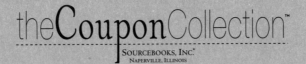

theCouponCollection™

SOURCEBOOKS, INC.
NAPERVILLE, ILLINOIS

take a
rest

Sit back on your heels, place your hands on your knees, and relax! Don't forget to breathe deeply!

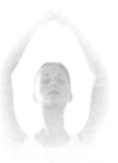

theCouponCollection™

SOURCEBOOKS, INC.
NAPERVILLE, ILLINOIS

Kundalini yoga

combines movement with breath. Try the frog pose and stretch your back and legs.

Start in a squat with your hands on the floor. As you inhale, straighten your legs so you're standing up and reaching for your toes. As you exhale, come back to a squat. Repeat four times, then rest.

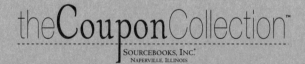

Bikram yoga

practices in a warm room for flexibility. Try putting on a few layers of extra clothing, or warm up the room as you stretch. See if you're more flexible when you're warm.

theCouponCollection

SOURCEBOOKS, INC.
NAPERVILLE, ILLINOIS

Iyengar yoga

focuses on the details of each posture. Try a warrior pose with perfect alignment.

Stand at the back of your mat, then step forward with your right foot. Rotate your left foot so you can put your heel on the floor. Bend your right knee exactly above your right ankle. Tuck your tailbone and raise your arms over your head. After a few breaths, repeat on the other side. Come back to standing when you're finished.

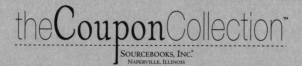

theCouponCollection™

SOURCEBOOKS, INC.
NAPERVILLE, ILLINOIS

Bhakti yoga

is service to others. Today help someone you love with a task or project.

theCouponCollection™

SOURCEBOOKS, INC.
NAPERVILLE, ILLINOIS

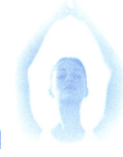

Raja yoga

is meditation. Take a few minutes to sit quietly and tune in to your breath. Empty your mind.

theCouponCollection™

SOURCEBOOKS, INC.
NAPERVILLE, ILLINOIS

take a **breath**

Use alternate nostril breathing to balance the two sides of the body.

Use your right thumb to close your right nostril, and inhale through your left nostril. Release your thumb and close your left nostril with the first two fingers of your right hand. Exhale through your right nostril. Close the left nostril and inhale through your right nostril, then close the right nostril and exhale through the left. Repeat for several cycles, then breathe normally for several breaths.

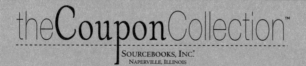

strike a pose

Try cobra pose for a classic stretch for the front of the body.

Lie on your belly on the floor. Place your forehead on the floor and your hands flat on the floor directly under your shoulders. Inhaling, lift your chin and chest slightly off the floor. Use your hands for balance, then press into them gently and come up just a few inches. Keep your elbows in close to your ribs. Exhaling, release the forehead back to the floor.

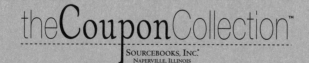

take a
rest

Do the alligator pose as a lovely way to relax!

Lying on your belly on the floor,
let your heels flop open and your big toes
touch. Place one hand over the other and rest
one cheek on top of your hands. After
a few breaths, switch hands and turn
your head to the other side.

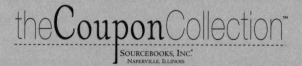

theCouponCollection™

SOURCEBOOKS, INC.
NAPERVILLE, ILLINOIS

strike a
pose

Stretch the whole body with the boat pose!

Lying on your belly on the floor, stretch your legs out behind you with big toes touching and your arms straight out in front of you with palms separated but facing each other. As you inhale, lift your arms, head, chest, and legs off the floor. Stretch your arms and legs as far as you can. On the exhale, release.

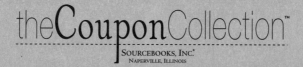

take a
rest

Enjoy the child's pose as a classic resting posture. Babies even sleep this way!

Sit back on your heels, lower your forehead to the floor, and relax. Arms can be stretched out in front, or alongside you on the floor.

theCouponCollection™

SOURCEBOOKS, INC.
NAPERVILLE, ILLINOIS

turn the world upside down!

Try an inverted posture for a new perspective on life!

Stand with your feet about four feet apart. Fold over and reach for your toes. Look at the world upside down! When you're ready to come up, stretch your arms out to the side and inhale your way up.

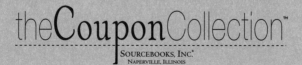

turn the world upside down!

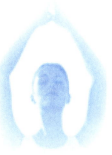

Do the downward dog!

Start on your hands and knees. Exhaling, straighten your knees and send your tailbone toward the ceiling. Press your armpits toward your knees and your heels toward the floor. Let your head relax. To finish, come back to your hands and knees.

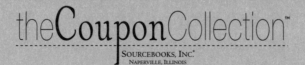

breath and movement **together**

Try a few Cat and Dog stretches to warm up your spine and connect you to your breath.

Start on your hands and knees.
As you inhale, tilt your tailbone to the ceiling and arch your back. Look up. As you exhale, tuck your tailbone under and round your spine like an angry cat. Tuck your chin. Repeat a few times, with your breath.

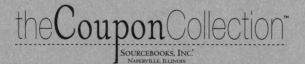

yoga
in a chair

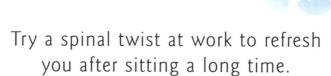

Try a spinal twist at work to refresh
you after sitting a long time.

Sit up straight in your chair with your feet flat on the floor. Twist to the right, reaching your left hand around to grasp the back of the chair. Turn your head to look over your right shoulder. Take a few breaths, then slowly rotate to the other side.

theCouponCollection™

SOURCEBOOKS, INC.
NAPERVILLE, ILLINOIS

yoga
in a chair

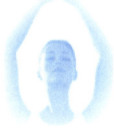

Link your breath and some movement to wake yourself up.

Sit up straight in your chair. As you inhale, circle your arms up over your head, and let your palms touch. As you exhale, circle your arms down. Repeat five to ten times. Keep your shoulders and neck relaxed.

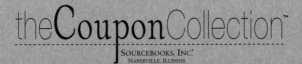

flex
your neck

Try a few neck rolls to relieve stiffness.

Sit up straight and gently lower your chin to your chest. Gently roll your chin over to your right shoulder, then back to center. Roll to the left, and return to center. Now lift your chin and look up at the ceiling. Roll to the right, then the left, and return your chin to center.

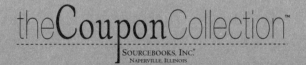

give your feet a
break

Do a few foot exercises to wake up tired feet.

Sitting on the floor with your legs stretched out in front of you, gently circle your ankles in one direction a few times, then in the other direction. Then alternately flex your feet and point your toes a few times.

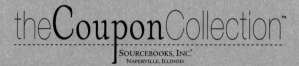

try a yoga **meal**

Eat a vegetarian lunch or dinner today. Try out a recipe, or visit a gourmet vegetarian restaurant. See if you feel lighter!

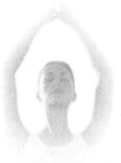

theCouponCollection™

SOURCEBOOKS, INC.®
NAPERVILLE, ILLINOIS

take a
rest

Whatever you're doing, close your eyes for a moment and take a few deep breaths.

You'll be amazed at how refreshed
you feel afterwards.

theCouponCollection™

SOURCEBOOKS, INC.
NAPERVILLE, ILLINOIS

watch a
video

Take a yoga video out of the library,
or rent one at your local video store.

You may learn brand new poses
that you've never done before.

theCouponCollection™

SOURCEBOOKS, INC.
NAPERVILLE, ILLINOIS

create a
yoga mood

Play some soft music and
burn a little incense.

Sit quietly in a comfortable cross-legged position and breathe deeply.

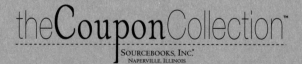

chant the sound of **om**

Breathe in deeply through your nose, and chant the universal sound of OM for the full length of your breath.

Try three repetitions—
chanting can be very soothing.

theCouponCollection™

SOURCEBOOKS, INC.
NAPERVILLE, ILLINOIS

strike a
pose

Do the Dancer pose to strengthen your balance.

Stand up straight. Bring all the weight onto your left foot and bend your right knee back. Take hold of the inside of your right ankle with your right hand and press the ankle into your hand to lift your leg behind you. Stretch your left hand straight out in front of you and lean forward a little. Focus your eyes on a spot on the floor about three feet ahead of you for balance. Come out of the posture with control, and try the other side.

theCouponCollection™

SOURCEBOOKS, INC.
NAPERVILLE, ILLINOIS

do yoga **outside**

Find a place where the ground is level,
and try a few postures.

You'll be amazed at how being outside in nature adds a new dimension to your yoga practice.

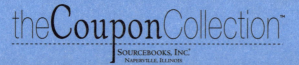

strike a **pose**

Do a few leg lifts at the end of your practice to help your legs relax.

Lie on your back with your palms flat on the floor. Flex your feet and gently lift your right leg to a 90-degree angle. Lower it slowly to about one inch from the floor, then lift it again. Do as many repeats as you'd like, then switch legs.

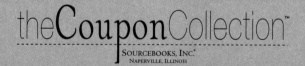

take a
breath

Do some breathing at the end of your practice to help your body integrate the postures.

Sit up straight in a comfortable cross-legged position. Breathe deeply and imagine the air traveling all the way up your spine as you inhale, and all the way down your spine as you exhale.

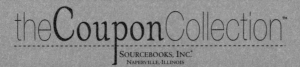

Relax!

Anytime you feel fatigued, do the Corpse pose.
It's like getting a good nap!

Lie on the floor with your arms at
your sides, palms facing up. Let your feet
flop open, and your entire body relax.
Stay here for a few minutes—five is ideal—
and see how refreshed you'll feel
when you get up.

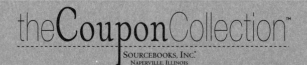

theCouponCollection™

SOURCEBOOKS, INC.
NAPERVILLE, ILLINOIS

∽ a gift for the spirit ∽

A Little Bit of Yoga: A Coupon Gift to Energize and Relax You

A Little Bit of Feng Shui: A Coupon Gift to Gently Shift Your Energies

Simple Serenity: A Coupon Gift to Help and Support You

Living in Abundance: A Coupon Gift to Enhance and Enrich You

Available at your local gift store or bookstore or by calling (800) 727-8866.

Collect them all!

∽ a breath of fresh air ∽

Going Over the Hill Slowly: A Coupon Gift That Keeps You Young
The Wild Side of Womanhood: A Coupon Gift to Unleash Your Audacious Power
Get a Grip: A Coupon Gift to Put You Back in Charge
The Goddess Within: A Coupon Gift that Celebrates You

∽ the country life ∽

I Love You Grandma: A Unique Tear-Out Coupon Gift of Love and Thanks
Dear Mom: A Unique Tear-Out Coupon Gift Just for You
Country Cat: A Unique Tear-Out Coupon Gift for the Feline Lover
A Country Life Wherever You Are: A Unique Tear-Out Coupon Gift for a Simpler Life

Available at your local gift store or bookstore or by calling (800) 727-8866.
Collect them all!

∽ from me to you ∽

I Love You Dad: A Coupon Gift of Love and Thanks
I Love You Mom: A Coupon Gift of Love and Thanks
Dear Grad: A Coupon Gift of Congratulations
Best of Friends: A Coupon Gift of Love and Thanks

∽ a drop of sunshine ∽

Slow Down: A Book of Peaceful Coupons
Faith, Hope and Love: A Coupon Gift to Restore Your Spirit
Angels: A Coupon Gift of Miracles
The Artist in You: A Coupon Gift to Spark Your Creativity

Available at your local gift store or bookstore or by calling (800) 727-8866.
Collect them all!

theCouponCollection™

SOURCEBOOKS, INC.®
NAPERVILLE, ILLINOIS